I0427858

A Guide to Staying Healthy Pregnancy and Your Baby
Understanding Pregnancy Symptoms
Staying Fit and Healthy throughout Your Pregnancy

By: Nillie Charles

A Guide to Staying Healthy Pregnancy and Your Baby

Understanding Pregnancy Symptoms Staying Fit and Healthy throughout Your Pregnancy

By: Nillie Charles

Table of Contents

Introduction

Congratulations, you're pregnant! As soon as you see the positive sign on the pregnancy test stick, you're sure to be feeling a myriad of emotions. Excitement, at the prospect of being a mother in nine months; trepidation, because you have no idea what to expect while you're pregnant; nervous, because you want what's best for you and your baby; and on top of all that, joyful as you think about welcoming this new addition to your family. If it's your first time being pregnant, know that these feelings are all normal and a lot of women have gone through this and felt the way you're feeling right now. Before we had access to all the information there is out there about pregnancy, women had to rely on well-meaning but sometimes outdated and inaccurate advice from loved ones about the things that should and should not be done while pregnant. One thing that everyone can agree on, from you, your OB Gyne, and your family, is that throughout your pregnancy, you should definitely take care of your health and that of your baby's well-being.

This book is a practical guide on how to be fit and healthy during pregnancy. In the first few chapters you'll know all about the symptoms of pregnancy and how to deal with the discomfort that comes with it. Then, read about the best food to eat while you're expecting, and what's safe to eat and drink for you and your baby. Choosing the right doctor is a must, and this book will also cover how to know if the doctor is the right one for you, as well as the tests and checkups which you'll do every month. Staying active while pregnant is important to have a healthy body and to prepare for the day when you'll be giving birth, so there's a chapter dedicated to exercise. Also, for those moms-to-be who are advised to go on bed rest, this book will show you how to cope with all the time that you have on your hands. Lastly, being healthy means that your whole physical, mental and emotional state is all in good order, so definitely making sure that you stay optimistic and cheerful is a must. And what girl doesn't feel happy when she looks good? The last two chapters will discuss how to look great while pregnant, with style and beauty tips for the expecting mom.

A few reminders before reading this book:
- If you're not sure what to do at any point in your pregnancy, call your OB Gyne and ask. At this point there is no such thing as a silly question, especially when it comes to you and your baby's health.
- Always have your monthly checkup to make sure that you and your baby are both doing well.
- Women have different experiences when it comes to pregnancy. Some lucky ones breeze through it with nothing more than a baby bump to show for it, while others seem to get all of the side effects of it, nausea, morning sickness, acne, aches and pains and other things aside from these. Never compare your pregnancy with that of another woman's pregnancy. Remember that we

are all made differently and what is true for you may not necessarily apply to her, and vice versa.

- Enjoy your pregnancy! It is an experience that you will never forget, so make it a happy one!

Pregnancy Symptoms

Some women experience all the typical symptoms of pregnancy, while others will only feel one or two. It's a different experience for each woman going through this, that's why it's important to know the different symptoms indicating pregnancy. Of course, you can drop by the drugstore and buy a pregnancy stick, but it's also important to listen closely to what your body is telling you. Once you're pregnant, it's important to be aware of the changes that your body is going through. After all, you won't be only taking care of yourself- there's a life inside of you that you have to care for too, starting with this crucial nine months.

Here are the typical symptoms of pregnancy:

1. *Aversion to certain smells*

   If you just found out or suspect that you're pregnant, you may find that certain food smells that used to appeal to you might be revolting all of a sudden. It's different for every woman, but some might be inclined to gag at the smell of onions and garlic being sautéed in the kitchen, or will flinch at the smell of brewing coffee, or even stop using her favorite perfume because the smell bothers her.

2. *Mood swings*

   Hormonal changes in the body during pregnancy triggers mood swings, so one minute you could be happy as a clam, the next you're enraged at the slightest provocation. Don't worry, this is normal. However if you're feeling sad, depressed or unable to manage your day to day responsibilities, contact a mental health professional for help.

3. *Bloating*
    Again, hormonal changes are responsible for this. Even at the earliest stages of pregnancy you will feel bloated, similar to what you feel before your period. Your clothes will feel a little tight around the waist, even though your uterus is still quite small.

4. *The urge to urinate more frequently*
    When you're pregnant, hormonal changes prompt a chain of activity in your body which causes an increase of blood flow through your kidneys, which makes your bladder fill up quickly, and makes you need to urinate frequently. This will continue as your pregnancy progresses, even more so as your growing baby exerts more pressure on your bladder.

5. *Feeling exhausted*
    If you often feel tired that all you want to do is take frequent naps all day long, it's your hormones again that are to blame. If you experience morning sickness and if you frequently have to get up at night to urinate, these could also contribute to the tired feeling you're experiencing.

6. *Sensitive, swollen breasts*
    The soreness and swelling might feel the same as when you're premenstrual, multiplied five times. The discomfort is temporary, and will soon get better after the first trimester.

7. *Nausea*

   Some women may experience morning sickness a month after conception, others may start having it a week or two earlier. Luckily, this will go away by the start of the second trimester. Morning sickness, despite the name, does not necessarily occur in the mornings only. It can be a problem morning, noon or night.

8. *You missed your period*

   It's easy to keep track of it especially if your period is pretty much regular, so if your period does not appear on time, you can take a pregnancy test even before some of the aforementioned symptoms happen.

9. *Basal body temperature is high*

   If you're trying to get pregnant and you notice that your basal body temperature stays high consistently for about 18 days, you're probably pregnant.

If you want to make sure, take a home pregnancy test. Most pregnancy test are not sensitive enough to indicate pregnancy hormones during the early days that you think you're pregnant, so it's best to wait after a week or so after you missed your period.
For someone who's pregnant for the first time, remember that all of these symptoms are normal and that there are ways to ease the discomfort that you feel.

Dealing with Discomfort

Pregnancy is a beautiful thing, but some of the things that come with it can be uncomfortable and annoying. Part of having a healthy pregnancy is learning how to deal with the discomfort that comes with it. This chapter aims to help you find safe and healthy ways to cope with the side effects of pregnancy such as morning sickness, constipation, hemorrhoids, itchy skin, and others. In the meantime, remember that all these symptoms are temporary and will be gone over time.

-Bleeding gums
If you find traces of blood when you brush your teeth, don't panic. Tender, swollen gums that are prone to bleeding is one of the most common complaints of pregnant women. Higher progesterone levels in your body makes your gums more sensitive to the plaque on your teeth, and this increases the blood supply to your mouth. In the meantime, switch to a toothbrush with soft bristles, and try not to floss too aggressively.

-Constipation
This affects other pregnant women too, so if any consolation, you're definitely not alone in this. This is caused by the slowed movement of food through your digestive tract, which is again caused by progesterone. To ease constipation, eat high-fiber foods such as whole grain cereals and breads, and make it a habit to have at least three servings of fruits and vegetables every day. Drink plenty of water, and never put off going to the bathroom when you feel like going.

-Hemorrhoids
Some women get hemorrhoids for the first time when they get pregnant. Hemorrhoids can be itchy or even painful and can cause rectal bleeding when making a bowel movement. Constipation can also cause hemorrhoids, so avoid getting constipated. If you do get hemorrhoids, apply an ice pack with a soft covering to the affected area several times a day. You can also try sitting in a warm sitz bath for 10 to 15 minutes a few times a day. Alternate cold and warm treatments throughout the day. Moisturizing the area can also help. Try using wipes medicated with witch hazel.

-Morning sickness
Ironically, most pregnant women get morning sickness not because of food smells, but because they're hungry. Make sure to have small snacks on hand to eat throughout the day. In fact, snacking is highly encouraged for pregnant women. Good snacks to have are cut up vegetables and fruits, Saltine crackers, and dried fruit and nuts. Also, avoid eating big meals.

-Itchy Skin
It's not uncommon for you to feel itchy around your belly and breasts, especially as your skin stretches to accommodate them. To soothe itchy skin, try applying some cocoa butter or unscented moisturizer on the affected area. You can also take a warm oatmeal bath once in a while. Wear loose clothing made from cotton. And, avoid going out during the hottest part of the day because heat can make the condition worsen.

-*Leg Cramps*

This happens because your leg muscles are tired from carrying around all your extra weight. If you get a cramp, have someone help you flex your toes by gripping them under and pushing. To prevent cramps from happening, don't sit for long periods of time with your legs crossed, and rotate your ankles whenever you're sitting. Stretch your legs by going for a walk every-day.

Great Food to Eat While You're Expecting

Some women who get pregnant the first time think that eating well means eating for two- sometimes more than that. However, it's not about the quantity but the quality of food that you ingest that matters. Remember that whatever you eat or drink can affect the health of your baby, so it's important to be mindful about what you put in your mouth.

What are the best foods to eat when you're expecting? Here is a partial list of those foods:

- **Salmon**- has Omega- 3fats and a great source of protein. Eat no more than 12 ounces a week to avoid ingesting too much mercury, though salmon is a low- mercury fish.
- **Beans**- these contain the most fiber out of all the vegetables which helps prevent constipation and hemorrhoids.
- **Sweet potatoes**- a great source of Vitamin C, folate and fiber. They're inexpensive and versatile so you can come up with many ways to prepare sweet potatoes before you get tired of eating them.
- **Whole grains**- feel free to indulge in popcorn, quinoa, oatmeal and whole grain bread. They're all high in protein and have many nutrients that will benefit both you and your baby.
- **Walnuts**- a handful of these omega-3 rich nuts make a good snack. Or chop up a few and add to a green salad to up the health factor.
- **Yoghurt**- it's very important to choose the right kind of yoghurt as there are a lot of choices out there, not to mention the proliferation of frozen yoghurt or froyo

stores. The best option for you is Greek yoghurt- it's thick, creamy and is high in calcium. Add some fresh fruit for flavor.

- **Dark green, leafy vegetables-** load up on spinach, kale, Swiss chard and the like for all the essential vitamins and minerals that are packed in each leaf. They're loaded with vitamins A, C and K and folate.

- **Lean meats-** look for lean meats with the fats trimmed off, or look for cuts that are at least 95 to 98 per cent fat free. Never eat deli meats or hot dogs unless they're heated until steaming hot, to prevent the risk of passing on toxins or bacteria to your baby such as salmonella.

- **Fruits and Vegetables-** as a guide on what to choose, look no further than the colors of the rainbow. Green, orange, red, yellow, purple, blue and even white fruits and veggies provide different vitamins and minerals. Another advantage of eating lots of these when you're expecting is, during the later stage of your pregnancy, your baby will be "tasting" the food through the amniotic fluid. So the earlier you expose the baby to a variety of healthy foods, the more you increase the chance that your baby will accept and like those foods later on.

- **Eggs-** aside from containing more than 12 vitamins and minerals, eggs are a good source of protein. They are rich in choline and there are some that even contain omega-3 fats. Eat eggs only if they're cooked thoroughly, such as hard boiled or scrambled.

What is Safe to Eat and Drink?

The ongoing debate about what are the safe foods to eat remain alive and well even through many generations. Blame it on old wives tales or unsolicited advice. But as an expecting mother, you should make it a point to be mindful of food and beverages that might affect you and your baby during pregnancy. As always, it's better to be safe than sorry. If you're unsure about whether something is safe or not, it's a good idea to ask your OB Gyne about it.

Here are the common questions that pregnant women ask :

1. *Is it safe to drink coffee while I'm pregnant?*

   Generally speaking, pregnant women and those who are trying to conceive should avoid drinking large quantities of caffeine. However, after decades of debates between medical experts, there's still no actual consensus on how much caffeine is safe during pregnancy. One thing's for sure though, if you stop drinking coffee, you won't feel jittery, you won't get an upset stomach, and the chances of getting heartburn is lessened, since caffeine is a major cause of it. You also ensure that your baby won't be born with a low birth weight. Be aware that caffeine comes in many forms, such as chocolate, tea, soft drinks, energy drinks and coffee ice cream.

2. *Is it safe to eat fish and other seafood while I'm pregnant?*

   Yes it is, but choose seafood that's low in mercury. A baby that's exposed to high levels of mercury can have developmental delays in the future, so make sure that the fish on your plate won't harm you or your baby. Among those that are in the safe to eat list are shrimp, scallops, flounder, sole, clams, tilapia, catfish, whitefish, king crab, crayfish and croaker. Those to avoid are king mackerel, shark, swordfish and tilefish. Vary the types of fish and seafood you eat during the course of the week so that you have only one serving of one kind, and no more than three servings of the same kind within the same week.

3. *Is it safe to drink herbal teas while I'm pregnant?*
   It depends on the type of tea. Avoid teas that contain any ingredients that can stimulate the uterus and induce a miscarriage such as anise, chamomile, comfrey, hibiscus, lemongrass, sage, sassafras and licorice root. Also avoid St. John's wort and kava tea because they have pharmacological actions. Among those that are safe to drink are peppermint and fresh ginger tea. Aside from being safe to drink, they also help curb nausea.

4. *Is it safe to eat spicy foods while I'm pregnant?*
   Yes, spicy food is safe to eat, but it might be uncomfortable for you if you make it a habit to eat highly-spiced foods. A lot of pregnant women suffer from heartburn, and if you're one of them, it's better if you avoid eating them altogether since spicy food aggravates heartburn.

5. *Is it safe to eat sushi while I'm pregnant?*
   No. Raw sushi may contain bacteria that can make you sick, as most raw fish harbor some parasites. Even the most careful among sushi chefs cannot get rid of all these

harmful bacteria. If you really have a craving for Japanese food, have some cooked sushi, make sure that it's cooked all the way through.

6. *Is it safe to have a glass of wine during dinner while I'm pregnant?*

No. Women who drink during pregnancy have an increased chance of giving birth to babies with Fetal Alcohol Syndrome, and a baby who has FAS is born smaller, and may have learning and behavioral problems.

7. *Is it safe to eat soft cheeses while I'm pregnant?*

It's only safe if you choose cheeses that are made using pasteurized milk. The ones you should avoid are the ones that are made with raw or unpasteurized milk such as feta, Brie, Camembert, Roquefort, gorgonzola, queso blanco, queso fresco, and panela.

8. *Is it safe to eat chocolate while I'm pregnant?*

It depends on the kind and quantity. Don't overdo it because you'll lose your appetite for other healthy foods and it can lead to excessive weight gain. If you have been diagnosed with gestational diabetes, you should avoid chocolate.

9. *Is it ok to eat salty foods while I'm pregnant?*

Unless you have high blood pressure, you don't need to worry about this. A moderate amount of sodium in the body is actually good for you because it can help maintain the fluid levels in your body.

10. *Is it ok to eat honey while I'm pregnant?*
    As long as the honey is pasteurized, it's safe to eat. Avoid eating raw honey because it can cause botulism, which is a form of food poisoning.

Prenatal Tests and Care

Aside from eating the right food, it's important to get proper care from a healthcare provider once you get pregnant. You will be prescribed the right vitamins to help you have a healthy pregnancy and help your baby develop well. You will also have to go through monthly checkups to make sure that everything is going well with your pregnancy, and to manage any complications that may arise while you're expecting.

Once you find out that you're pregnant, you'll need to find a physician whom you trust and feel comfortable with. Choosing a doctor will depend on you, and if some well-meaning relative recommends a doctor whom you feel is not the right fit for you, you have every right to find another. You and your doctor will be seeing a lot of each other for the next 9 months and even beyond that for post natal care. Most women prefer a female doctor because they feel that they can truly empathize with what they're going through, and in the end it is just more comfortable that way.

What is a good doctor like? First, the doctor must have a caring, sincere and empathic attitude. If a doctor genuinely cares about you and your baby's well being, then she will pay more attention to your symptoms and keep on finding solutions when a particular treatment is not effective. A good doctor will also take the time to answer all the questions that you have. Some women will think that just because a particular physician has a long line outside her office, then she must be "the one". However, keep in mind that sometimes, the more patients a doctor has, the less quality time she can allot to each one.

Once you find the right doctor, he or she will recommend that you undergo a couple of basic prenatal tests. Now don't be anxious about these tests as these are one of the many ways to check on your well being and that of your growing baby. At your first prenatal test, your OB will give you a physical, and that includes a pelvic exam. A Pap smear will be done to rule out any abnormal cells, unless you've already had one done recently. Next, routine blood tests will be done to check your blood type and Rh status, and a blood count to check for anemia. The lab will also test your blood for Syphilis, Hepatitis B, immunity to German measles and chicken pox. If you are a high risk for gestational diabetes then you'll also get tested for that.

You should get a monthly checkup during the duration of your pregnancy. During these checkups you will be weighed to see if you're gaining weight (which is normal, by the way) and how fast you're gaining. A Doppler will also be used to check your baby's heartbeat. On your 6th to 10th week of pregnancy you will have an ultrasound to confirm the date of the pregnancy, thus enabling your doctor to calculate your due date. On the fifth month you'll have another sonogram to measure your baby's size, check the location of the placenta, check for physical abnormalities, and find out the baby's gender.

Exercising and Staying Active While Pregnant

When a woman gets pregnant for the first time, most people will try to tell her to take it easy and get lots of rest. This advise is quite easy to follow, since pregnancy will make you feel like taking a nap every now and then, and snacking while "taking it easy" in front of the TV. However, it's still important to remain active and do some form of exercise while pregnant. Though training for the next marathon is not in the cards for most moms-to-be, there are other exercises that will benefit you and your baby. The days when it was thought that exercise could lead to miscarriage are over. Except for really high risk situations, pregnant women are now encouraged to participate in some low impact exercises. By doing so, this can   help in making them feel well, both physically and mentally.

Aside from helping you feel great, what are the other benefits you can get if you exercise while you're pregnant? For one thing, you'll gain less unnecessary weight. You'll also be less likely to develop stretch marks and your body will bounce back to its pre-baby shape more quickly. Moms-to-be who are reasonably active experience less fatigue and nausea than moms who are living the sedentary life. You'll also prevent common pregnancy related health issues such as back aches, heart burn, constipation, bloating and swelling. Finally, women who exercise moderately during pregnancy experience less pain during labor.

Now, before you think about logging in hours at the gym, you've got to know how much time is enough time for exercise now that you're pregnant. Thirty minutes a day is enough to feel good and get all the benefits from staying active. So, keeping that in mind, here are a few exercises that you can do:

- **Yoga**- though you won't be able to do the usual poses you've done prior to getting pregnant, you should be able to keep up and modify the poses when you need to do so. Even better, take a prenatal yoga class. If there is nowhere near you that offers this type of class, you can browse the internet for videos.

- **Strength training**- it's not about lifting weights, it's more about body weight exercises. Do some squats, lunges, planks, bridges, push-ups, and dips. These exercises help tone and tighten various parts of the body. If you do decide to do some weight lifting, use lightweight dumbbells, ideally no more than 1 pound weights on each hand and do more repetitions. Do not lift more than 5 pounds per hand.

- **Light aerobic activity**- light means light. Now is not the time to break out the Zumba moves. Instead, do some light walking, swimming, or dancing without fast, jerky movements.

There will be days when you don't feel like working out, and those kinds of days outnumber the days when you feel fine. Whenever that happens, it's important to listen to your body and trust your instincts. If you feel exhausted or crampy anywhere in your body, it's ok to rest and exercise on another day.

Coping with Bed Rest

There are two reactions that naturally occur when the words "bed rest" are mentioned. Some pregnant women may sigh with relief, happy to be off their feet and spend their pregnancy in bed. Others might feel depressed, scared and bored. If you were advised by your doctor to go on bed rest, don't despair. There are things that you can do to prepare for the arrival of your little one without leaving the comfort of your bedroom.

What are the reasons why doctors may prescribe bed rest? Doctors will urge you to do bed rest for a prescribed period of time if you have high blood pressure, placenta previa, or if you're having twins or multiples, experience frequent spotting or bleeding, contractions or any signs of preterm labor. Discuss the things that you can do, and more importantly, the things that you are not allowed to do. There are some cases wherein expectant mothers are not allowed to leave the bed at all, and some are allowed to go as far as the bathroom and all other parts of the home provided that there will be no need to climb stairs.

Here are a couple of things that you can do to cope with bed rest:
- *Stay connected to your family and friends*

  Are you missing out on major family events or a friend's birthday or wedding because you were told to go on bed rest? Being on bed rest can make you feel isolated from the rest of the world since you may not be allowed to walk around or even get out of the house. But you don't have to spend your pregnancy sulking because you couldn't have a good time with your loved ones. Stay connected to them by encouraging them to visit you, or talk to you on the phone.

- *Look for an online support group if you have a laptop or Android tablet.*
  You might be surprised to find out that you are not alone in this and that some other mom-to-be out there is having a more difficult time than you. Here's the chance to make new friends, to get and offer words of encouragement from other women.

- *Opt to work from home*
  You vowed to yourself that you would be the kind of pregnant woman who can still work and juggle pregnancy at the same time. If taking an extended leave of absence is not an option for you, ask your employer if it's possible for you to work from home. Since many things can be done over the internet and the phone, this might be a good arrangement for you. Just make sure to let your boss know the things your physician specifically said you can do, so that all of you are on the same page, without putting you, your baby, and your job at risk.

- *Make like a Girl Scout and always be prepared.*
  Before your spouse or family head out the door each day, make sure that you get help from them preparing all the things you need before they leave. Have a fully charged phone on your bedside table, and a list of emergency numbers that you can call, including your doctor's

number. Make sure that you have something to eat and drink within arm's reach, and a change of clothes and underwear on the bed should you happen to need them. Keep the TV and DVD remote near you, and other materials to while the time away such as books, magazines, or crafting materials.

- *Take advantage of all this free time*
  Now is the time for you to watch the TV shows and movies that you've always wanted to watch, and read the books that you never had time to read until now. Once you have the baby, free time will definitely become a thing of the past.

- *Do some light organization*
  Now is the best time to do some light organization, such as sorting the documents In your laptop into specific folders. You can also start a journal if you like.

- *Shop online*
  Do you get frustrated that you'll miss out on the fun of picking out your baby's things because you can't go to the mall? Relax. Got your laptop and credit card? There's always online shopping.

Lastly, remember why you're doing this. It might be inconvenient and frustrating at times, but in the end, it's worth it once you get to hold your baby in your arms.

How Have Style While Pregnant

Aside from being physically fit, it's also important to be emotionally healthy while you're pregnant. Most women tend to feel depressed as their bodies grow to accommodate the baby. Some women seem to look pregnant only from a lateral view- you know the type, those women who only look pregnant from the side. And there are some who seem to gain weight everywhere else. When this happens, most expectant mothers feel frustrated because nothing seems to fit, and everything looks awkward. Pregnancy is overwhelming, and transforming your wardrobe will seem like a challenge. But you don't have to spend money on maternity clothes that you'll only wear for a few months. Here are several wardrobe adjustments you can make, secrets to pregnancy dressing, as well as some pieces that you can incorporate into your wardrobe that will enhance the natural glow that you've got:

1. During your first trimester, you might not need pregnancy pants yet. However, are your jeans starting to feel a little snug? Here's a trick that you can do up until your fourth month: Loop a hair elastic or a rubber band through the buttonhole of your jeans, and secure around the button. Wear a loose shirt over it, or an empire waist blouse.

2. Consider borrowing before you buy. Maternity clothes can be quite expensive, especially considering the fact that you'll only be wearing them for a few months. The more you can borrow from your friends or relatives who have been pregnant before, the better.

3. Shop your partner's closet for outfit possibilities. His oxford shirts can be worn unbuttoned over a tank or form fitting tee.

4. Wear leggings. They're comfortable, plus they can accommodate your growing belly. Stay away from leggings with a not-too-stretchy waistband, as this can pinch uncomfortably.

5. Long fitted shirts over leggings or jeans will show off your baby bump. Empire waist tops are good for balancing your figure. Thin knitwear works well for your shape.

6. When you purchase your first pair of maternity jeans, make sure to choose one with an adjustable waistband, a stretchy material, and a flattering cut that you can wear with cute and comfy flats. Consider buying one with a light wash for everyday wear, and another with a dark wash for special occasions.

7. The wrap dress is a blessing for most pregnant women. Diane Von Furstenberg makes the best ones. If you find that the wrap dress bares too much of your cleavage, you can wear a bandeau under it.

8. As your tummy gets bigger, you'll find that your shoes begin to feel a bit tighter. Wear comfy flats or any kind of slip on shoes. Avoid anything with laces- you do not want to be bending over to tie them. Now is also not the time to break out the high heels because pregnancy affects your

center of gravity, and your balance becomes a bit more precarious. If you really insist on heels, go for kitten heels or wide chunky heels.

9. Accessorize! Well-chosen accessories can elevate a plain outfit to something special. Wear a few bracelets and a watch on the same arm. Or choose a scarf to complement your outfit. Wear some fun earrings too.

10. While you're adding a few pieces to your wardrobe, make sure that you buy some new underwear too. Go for the comfy, full panties instead of the sexy lingerie- you'll feel better in it. You will definitely need new bras as your breasts will have gone up a cup size or two. Make sure that everything is made from breathable fabric to avoid itching.

Staying Pretty Throughout Pregnancy

Ever wonder how some celebrities go through pregnancy looking fresh faced and absolutely glowing? Take for instance, the Duchess of Cambridge, Kate Middleton. The woman simply glowed and was the picture of health. And of course, who could forget how a very pregnant Natalie Portman looked when she won an Oscar? She was radiant! Beyonce still looked fierce while pregnant with her baby, Blue Ivy. Ang Angelina Jolie looked perfect even while carrying twins Knox and Vivienne. Because these women have to look good at all times, they have people who are dedicated to making sure that they stay that way, even through pregnancy. As for the rest o us, we have ourselves to rely on to present our best face to the rest of the world.

Though it's hard to think about swiping on some mascara when you're dealing with morning sickness, a girl's gotta do what a girl's gotta do. We're not talking about a full face of makeup, just some little touches here and there that can boost a pregnant lady's confidence even when she's not feeling well. You'll be surprised how looking good can help you feel good. Also, you might need to tweak your beauty regimen a little to make sure that anything you put on your hair or body will not have adverse effects on your baby.

Let's do a checklist, from head to toe:

<u>Hair</u>

Your hair is probably looking its best right now. All that folic acid in your prenatal vitamins is behind that thick and shiny head of hair that you have. If you're bothered by the re-growth of hair after a dye job, you'll be happy to know that it's perfectly safe to color your hair. Studies have shown that there are not enough chemicals in the dye that can be absorbed into the blood stream through the scalp which can harm your baby. If you're still nervous about it, wait until the second trimester to color your hair. As for shampoo, try Aveda as all their shampoos have very little chemicals.

<u>Face</u>

You might have to adjust your skin care regimen a little while you're pregnant. If you're prone to acne, don't take Accutane for it since this can cause birth defects. Also, creams that have Vitamin A in them such as Retin-A should be avoided at this time. For now, switch to more natural and gentler options for your skin. Wash with a mild cleanser such as Cetaphil, and moisturize. Make sure to wear sunscreen whenever you go out. To treat pimples, dab a tea tree oil stick on it such as the Tea Tree Oil Stick from The Body Shop.

<u>Teeth</u>

If you're teeth are looking a bit yellowy, it's best to wait until the baby is born before you get your teeth bleached. Though there's no evidence that proves that the peroxide in the bleach can harm your baby, most dentists will strongly advise you to wait until you've given birth.

Body

Cleansing with any soap and moisturizing with an unscented lotion is the ideal everyday regimen for your body skin. Steer clear of any chemical hair removers and self tanning lotions while pregnant. Waxing is also safe, though you may find that it's more painful for you because you're pregnant.

Manicures and Pedicures

All perfectly safe to do. Just make sure to instruct your nail technician to use very light pressure when it's time to do the massage prior to applying the nail polish, because they might press on certain acupressure points which could induce labor. It's also a good idea to bring your own tools to minimize the risk of getting an infection. Pick nail polishes free of the "toxic 3", namely phthalate, toluene, and formaldehyde. Try these brands: Knocked Up Nails, which are made especially for pregnant women; Zoya, which has over 300 colors to choose from; and Piggy Paint, which was originally formulated with little kids in mind but now has a series of colors for expectant moms. Also, use non-acetone nail polish remover such as the soy-based nail polish remover from Scotch Naturals.

Makeup

Go ahead, put on some makeup, even on the days when you don't feel like it. In fact, especially on the days when you don't feel like it. Nothing will make you feel worse than looking into the mirror and seeing a blotchy complexion, dark shadows under your eyes, and pale cheeks and lips. You can keep on using the brands that you enjoy because the chances of the makeup affecting the baby are slim to none. At the very least, smooth on a tinted moisturizer or BB Cream (Laura Mercier and Smashbox have the best ones), some undereye concealer, a touch of finishing powder, some lip and cheek cream for a hint of rosy color (Stila has something called convertible color that's great for cheeks and lips), a few swipes of mascara, and ta-da! Instant pretty!